MILITARY DIET FOR BEGINNERS

A Simple Guide on how to live a healthy life and lose weight with the military diet

By

Dr. Tee Stevens

Copyright edition @ 2024

Contents

PREFACE

This book on Military diet will particularly teach you on how to lose weight effectively with the military diet. The book will simply guide you on how the military diet works, the military diet and the foods to consume on the diet, the military diet and the foods to avoid on the diet, the military diet and the potential benefits as well as the risks associated with the diet, the military diet and a 3-day meal plan and so many more.

INTRODUCTION

The military diet which is also referred to as the 3-day diet is a restrictive periodic fasting eating plan that may promote short-term loss of weight. It is a short-term diet that may be hard and potentially not safe to sustain. The military diet which claims to help lose up to 10 pounds in 7 days (1 week) is not related or associated with the military irrespective of its name. When individuals think of the word *"military"*, they might think of a strict regimen that involves both mental and physical strength, although there is no boot camp needed with this kind of diet. Amazingly, there is no exercise requirement whatsoever, although proponents do encourage day to day walks.

The military diet plan comprises of a 3-day, calorie-restricted plan accompanied by 4 days off (returning to regular eating for 4 days). Daily calorie intake is constricted to 1,400, 1,200 and 1,100 across the first 3 days while it is recommended you keep your calories below 1,500 for the 4 *"off"* days.

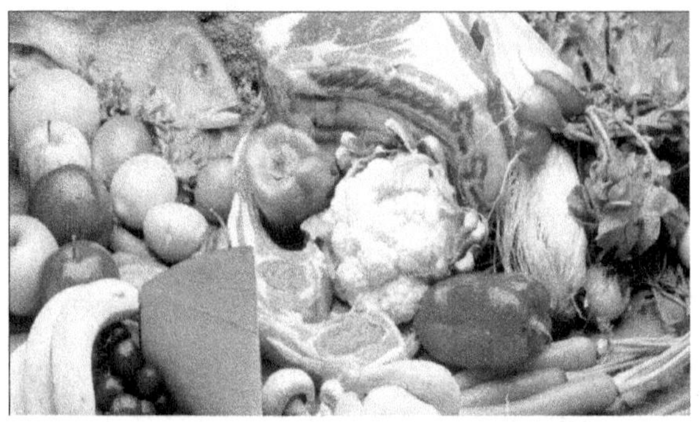

The food and drug administration recommends adults consume an average of 1,600 to 3,000 calories each day, subject to age and activity levels.

It is possible to iterate the cycle for up to a month, or until you attain your weight loss goal or objective.

Some individuals may decide to follow the military diet for longer terms (like iterating the diet with 4-days in between), although restricting your calories that extremely over a long duration of time is not healthy.

The military diet which is high in protein and low in fat, carbohydrate and calories involves specific food combinations to try to enhance metabolism and burn fat.

Advocates of the military diet affirms that the 3-days on and 4 *"off"* days method is effective enough to help you in losing weight with disrupting with your metabolism (a problem noticed on longer-term, extremely restrictive diets). Nevertheless, there is no assurance that you won't yield to food cravings at certain point during the three (3) days you are on the diet plan.

The military diet approves this eating plan for *"emergency situations"* where individuals *"need to shed unwanted pounds instantly."* It only appears to work for individuals who are capable of sticking with few calories and are able to fight the hunger and low energy that comes with it.

On the brighter side, the military diet is comparatively cheap and affordable since you are consuming real foods. The military diet plan does not require you to buy any processed foods, supplements as well as beverages.

Nevertheless, as soon as the low-calorie period is over, the effects of consuming more calories are likely to come back with a reprisal. For most individuals, following or adhering to the military diet is extremely hard and it can also be argued that a low calorie diet is just not realistic or sustainable.

Furthermore, if you are over the age of 50, very low-calorie diets could be hazardous and this is according to the

***National institute of Diabetes and Digestive and Kidney Diseases.**

There may be currently no intense studies on the military diet, although a calorie deficit is typically needed to achieve loss of weight, the military diet does not consider other factors that could influence weight loss such as genetics, sleeping habits, taking some medications, lifestyle habits as well as underlying health conditions.

A 2018 outline indicates that a calorie deficit of 500 to 600 calories is a feasible way to lose 0.5kg per week and for adult males, this is about 1,500 to 1,800 daily calories and for adult females, it is about 1,200 to 1,500.

These mild calorie restrictions are the reverse of the military diet's heavy restrictions.

A 2017 outline deduced that mild and sustained calorie restriction is just as effectual for weight loss as intermittent high energy restrictions, such as 3 days on and 4 days off.

Advocates of the military diet affirm that the specific food combinations in the meal plan increase your metabolism and burn excess fat, although there is no proven research to support these assertions.

Caffeine may be one component of the military diet that could aid in promoting body weight and loss of excess fat.

With regards to the safety of the diet, the military diet is unbalanced and repeating the cycle multiple times could result into health conditions such as nutrient deficiencies.

A 2014 outline and review indicates that substantial calorie reductions even for short term or short periods, such as in the case of the military diet may create or aggravate eating patterns, poor relationships with food, or disordered eating pattern.

Frequently consuming processed foods such as *hot dogs, crackers, and ice cream* has been associated with various health conditions such as *cardio-metabolic risks, obesity, cardiovascular diseases, depression, irritable bowel syndrome, cancer, and type 2 diabetes.*

A healthy eating pattern should comprise of whole and minimally processed foods such as legumes, beans, nuts, whole grains, fruits, vegetables, poultry, lean meat, seafood, and low or non-fat dairy products.

The military diet does not encourage positive long-term habitual changes and that entails that any weight that is lost can be instantly regained as soon as you return to your habitual eating regimen.

Establishing pragmatic weight loss goals and aiming for lifestyle changes instead of short-term fad diets is vital for remarkable weight loss, weight maintenance, and the prevention of weight regain.

Nevertheless, there have been no research or study to verify its claimed benefits and intense calorie restrictions may give rise to health problems.

CHAPTER ONE

THE MILITARY DIET AND HOW IT WORKS

The military diet makes numerous assertions, such as the promise that you will lose 10 pounds in 1 week (7 days). Nevertheless, everyone is different, and every individual loses weight in several ways and at contrasting rates. Always speak to your physician before attempting a new diet, particularly one that bans food groups or cut down on calories to a tiny number.

The military diet is an extremely strict, low-calorie diet with certain foods that appear healthy and others that don't seem healthy. There are set of foods to consume for breakfast, lunch as well as dinner. There are no snacks and there is no flexibility about food selections or choices based on your tastes.

The 3-day military diet is split into two (2) phases over the course of one week (7 days) and during the initial/first phase of 3 days; the total calorie intake is about 1,100 to 1,400 calories each day thus making it a low calorie diet, defined as a dietary pattern that provides 800 to 1,200 calories each day.

The military diet plan does allow 100 additional calories for men each day "ideally in the form of protein, and not carbs."

The military diet basically encourages individuals to follow and adhere to a 1,500 calorie diet. The military diet plan also opine that you can iterate the program as often as you would want to, if you would like to lose extra weight, in as much you take 4-day breaks every time after you do it.

It is vital to understand that this kind of *calorie restriction* falls below the approved daily calorie intakes of 2,200 to 2,400 for adult males and 1,600 to 1,800 for adult females.

Furthermore, before making any extreme restrictions, it is vital to consult a healthcare professional or a dietician. Not consuming sufficient calories may result into a wide range of **health conditions and health problems.**

CHAPTER TWO

THE MILITARY DIET AND FOODS TO CONSUME ON THE DIET

The military diet is a diet plan that affirms to be an instant way to lose weight by adhering to a strict diet, stating you will lose up to 10 pounds in 7 days (one week). For the first or initial 3 days, you adhere or follow a specific diet, which includes *hard-boiled eggs, coffee, cheddar cheese, and saltine crackers.* The diet plan recommends you continue to restrict or limit your calorie count on your 4 *"off"* days.

Every fragment you will consume on the military diet has already been chosen, and thus, you will just need to follow the plan completely to get the best and effective results.

Foods to consume on the military diet

(a) Bananas

(b) Apples

(c) Coffee

(d) Cheeses (cheddar and cottages), in small proportions

(e) Eggs (*Hard-boiled eggs*).

(f) Bread (whole-wheat), in small proportions

(g) Greek yogurt

(h) Green beans

(i) Peanut butter

(j) Meat

(k) Tea

(l) Tuna

(m) Ice-cream (vanilla ice-cream).

(n) Saltine crackers

(o) Hot dogs

(p) Grapefruit

(q) Carrots

(r) Broccoli

CHAPTER THREE

THE MILITARY DIET AND FOODS TO AVOID ON THE DIET

Limited substitutions are permitted on the Military diet plan in as much as meals stay within the calorie guidelines for the first three (3) days. The remaining 4*"off"* days, individuals are advised to eat or consume 1,500 calories each day of a less restrictive diet, preferably choosing healthier, whole foods over processed foods. Nevertheless, there are some foods to avoid on the military diet and they include:

(a) Dairy products *such as cream (in coffee), and milk.*

(b) Alcohol such as beer, wine, and spirits

(c) Sugar such as honey, maple syrup, agave, and white or brown sugar.

(d) Fruit juices

(e) Oranges

(f) Yogurt (aside from Greek varieties)

(g) Butter

(h) Artificial sweeteners (aside from stevia)

You can also adhere or follow the military diet if you are a vegetarian or vegan by replacing meats with *tofu or beans.*

It is vital to understand that many of the recommended or approved foods are low in fiber and thus, may go against most standard advice for weight loss. For instance, including high-fiber foods help you in keeping full without additional calories as outlined by the *American Heart Association.*

CHAPTER FOUR

THE MILITARY DIET AND ITS BENEFITS

The amount of weight that any individual can lose on a diet relies on various factors such as *age, genetics, gender, the extent of the calorie deficit as well as the amount of excess weight.*

For instance, people with a history of obesity may lose weight much faster than individuals currently at a healthy body weight. Typically speaking, it is more challenging to lose body fat if you are already within a healthy weight range.

Furthermore, it is common to observe quick weight loss at the beginning of a new diet, which may slow down or elevate as you attain your goal weight. It is vital to consider personal factors in order to set a weight loss objective that is rational and accomplishable. Numerous individuals find that their willpower slips when they set an objective that turns out to be unachievable.

A sustainable weight loss of around 3% to 5% from starting weight has the capability to enhance health by reducing the risk factors of heart disease and diabetes.

The military diet which basically focuses on protein may be beneficial in the short-term. The military diet is simple to follow since it includes limited foods with effortless measurements and cooking techniques.

The approved meal plan for the 4 *"off"* days allows for a wide range of vegetables and fruits, and it also comprises of whole grains, legumes and several meal options.

The military diet plan provides the calorie targets for each food and recommends replacement for individuals with *food intolerances* and other dietary considerations.

The military diet

- Increases the feeling of fullness
- Provides energy for daily activities
- Helps in maintaining muscle tissue as it directly contributes to an individual's metabolism.

A 2018 research analyzed the effects of following a diet with calorie restrictions on different days. The researchers examined the results of the diet with those of exercise in individuals with obesity.

In the participants who were both following or adhering to the military diet and exercising, body weight, waist circumference, and body fat percentage all reduced.

A 2016 research which examined a very low calorie diet with an alternate day fasting deduced that alternate day fasting was more effective for fat loss and preserving fat-free mass, such as *muscle.*

As a result of the military diet's approved daily calorie intake of 1,100 to 1,400 on the first or initial 3 days, it is not feasible to group it as either a very low calorie diet or an alternate day fasting program. Research and study on very low calorie diet or an alternate day fasting regimens only focuses at diets providing fewer than 800 calories each day.

In spite of the fact that calorie intake on the military diet is very high to count as fasting, the approach of eating normally on the 4 *"off"* days emulates the practice of *intermittent fasting.* Thus, individuals may achieve better long-term results by adhering or following this diet instead of a low-calorie diet.

A systematic review that examined successful strategies for weight loss among healthy adults deduced that, overall; a calorie deficit is required in order to produce remarkable weight loss. And due to the fact that the military diet is a low-calorie meal plan, it will presumably result into loss of weight by creating a calorie deficit.

Nevertheless, it is also deduced that a combination of calorie restriction, frequent exercise, and healthy behavior change was required to maintain this loss of weight. This could entail that adopting healthy habits is a more feasible approach for keeping the weight off than a short-term, instant fix diet such as the military diet menu.

Additional research is required to confirm any particular benefits of the military diet and how it helps to sustain healthy habits and maintain weight loss.

CHAPTER FIVE

MILITARY DIET AND ITS POTENTIAL RISKS

The biggest short-term risks associated with the military diet are constipation and binge-eating (due to over-restricting). When restricting some foods, you are likely to put yourself at risk of losing out some nutrients, which is something a multivitamin can't completely replace. The diet recommends as few as 1,100 calories each day, although most individuals will require at least 1,200 calories each day to meet bare minimum nutritional requirements.

Diets with intense calorie restrictions such as those touted by the military diet have also been connected to binge eating and eating disorders such as anorexia.

When you do extremely strict *"on" and "off"* diets such as the military diet, it can start to deform your view of food and if you have to avoid some foods completely, or can only follow a very specific diet, you are at risk of developing disordered eating which is an unhealthy relationship with food. And since a restrictive calorie diet isn't feasible, you will ultimately go back to eating normally and when your body has been in a *"scarcity"* mode, it will hang on to any energy it acquires, resulting into weight gain (what you lost on the diet and sometimes even more).

In a 2016 research from the American Academy of Pediatrics that tracked individuals between the ages of 14 and 15, it was deduced that those practicing diets with intense calorie restrictions were 18 times more presumably to develop an eating disorder than individuals who did not diet.

The poor variety on the military diet days means that individuals will struggle to consume sufficient fiber, minerals and vitamins. These nutrients are important for excellent health, energy production, detoxification, and proper metabolism.

The military diet may be high in added salt, sugar and saturated fat. Between the saltine crackers, cheddar, bread, hot dogs, cheese, and peanut butter, the military diet is somewhat high in processed foods that comprise of salt. Individuals should check nutrition labels to ensure that they are not consuming more sodium than the approved 2,300 milligrams a day limit. Where feasible, it is best to purchase food brands that are low in sodium or contain no added salt.

Vanilla ice cream which can be high in added sugar is also included in each day's meal plan. Individuals could alternate the ice-cream for 300 calories of healthy fruit, whole grains or vegetables which the plan basically lacks.

A diet that highlights high-calorie, dense foods may not feel extremely satisfying since portion sizes must remain small to keep meals within the day to day calorie budget. This approach may not be viable.

Consuming fewer than 1,400 calories on diet days may make it hard to perform exercise, particularly any high-intensity activities.

Note that the military diet does not include snacks, and thus you may feel hungry for long duration of time which could eventually drain your willpower.

Consuming sufficient calories on the 4 *"off"* days will permit individuals to exercise more easily, although advocates of the military diet recommend sticking to fewer than 1,500 calories on these days also.

A small research looking at alternate day calorie restriction also referred to as **intermittent fasting,** deduced that combining alternate day calorie restriction with exercise resulted into greater weight alterations than either dieting or exercise alone.

Following or adhering to a very low calorie diet can prevent individuals from exercising completely.

The military diet indicates that individuals who dislike or cannot eat **grapefruit** replace it for a glass of water with baking soda in it to continue to foster an alkaline environment.

It is proven that foods can change pH from acid to alkaline, although this mainly affects the acidity or alkalinity of an individual's urine. The pH of foods in the diet does not affect an individual's blood or metabolism enough to remarkably influence weight gain or weight loss, though it may affect other aspects of health.

All fruit give rise to alkaline byproducts in the body and as a result, replacing one fruit with another fruit should be ok.

The high-protein aspect of the diet will make urine more acidic and as a result, it may not be ideal for an individual experiencing *gout or kidney disease.*

The military diet lacks variety and calories during the diet period and as a result of the intense calorie restriction, most individuals will not eat enough fiber, healthy fat, vitamins and other essential nutrients during the 3-diet days.

For instance, the 3-day diet menu is significantly low in healthy fats, such as avocados and olive oil with studies demonstrating that a diet rich in heart-healthy monounsaturated fats, such as those found in olive oil may help in decreasing the risk of heart disease, particularly when used in place of saturated fat.

Furthermore, this menu depends on many of the same foods during the diet days, which may accidentally leave numerous healthy foods such as cabbage, spinach, strawberries, cauliflower, and leafy greens out of the diet.

CHAPTER SIX

THE MILITARY DIET AND A 3-DAY MEAL PLAN

The military diet does not ask you to avoid dairy products, carbs, or other food classes and again, you may not want to eat out when you are on the program, though, since the food choices are extremely strict, and you perhaps won't find them on a normal menu.

While it is an excellent idea to exercise each day, don't put much pressure on yourself by running or lifting heavy weights during the 3 days you are on this low-calorie diet. Light exercise such as gentle yoga or walking is fine.

The military diet 3-day meal plan typically comprises of 16 foods to be divided between breakfast, lunch, and dinner.

	Day 1	Day 2	Day 3

Breakfast	1 slice of whole-grain toast 1 tablespoon peanut butter ½ grapefruit 1 cup of tea without sugar or milk	1 slice of whole-grain toast 1 egg ½ banana 1 cup of coffee or tea 1 slice of cheddar cheese	1 slice cheddar cheese 1 apple 5 saltine cracker 1 cup of coffee
Lunch	1 toast ½ cup of tuna 1 cup of tea or black coffee	1 hard-boiled egg 1 cup cottage cheese 5 saltine cracker	1 toast 1 hard-boiled egg 1 cup of carrot 1 cup of

		s 1 cup of tea or coffee	coffee
Dinner	1 apple 1 cup vanilla ice cream 3 oz (ounces) meat 1 cup green beans ½ banana	½ cup carrots ½ cup vanilla ice-cream ½ cup banana ½ cup broccoli 2 hot dogs	1 cup vanilla ice-cream 1 cup tuna ½ banana 1 cup of broccoli

The military diet allows drinking water, herbal teas and caffeinated coffee or tea twice each day with no creamers or sugars.

There are no guidelines for the remaining 4 days of the military diet apart from adhering or following a **healthy eating regimen.**

For individuals who hope to speed up their weight loss even much more, a 1,500 calorie menu is available. For example, snacks are allowed during these days, although you are advised to **reduce your portion sizes.**

Note that consuming 1,500 calories each day is still a calorie restriction that may not fit everyone's energy requirements and this is particularly true if you lead an active lifestyle, which translates into increased energy expenditure and greater calorie requirements.

It is recommended that people following the 3-day diet plan drink enough water all through the day to promote proper hydration. You can as well sip on unsweetened black coffee or tea in as much as these beverages do not contain added calories from sugar, cream, or milk.

Sweeteners and most artificial sweeteners apart from Stevia in coffee are not permitted on the menu, which entails that soda and other sugary beverages will not work on the Military diet plan.

Typically, it is an excellent idea to drink water, black coffee, and unsweetened tea such as green, black and herbal teas.

The military diet permits substitutions during the 3-day phase, in as much as portions match the calorie count and these substitutions may be **lactose-free, gluten-free, vegan, vegetarian, and allergy-free.**

The military diet accentuates not substituting grapefruits for oranges but rather, it recommends substituting or replacing grapefruit with a glass of water with ½ teaspoon of baking soda. This is claimed to help alkalinize your body and decrease body fat.

Furthermore, vegans or vegetarians can replace meat or tuna with cottage cheese, tofu or tofu dogs, avocado, almonds or hummus.

Nevertheless, research demonstrates that while certain foods increase your body's acid load, your kidneys can excrete the excess acid via urine and thus, your dietary choices or options have small impact on your body's level of alkalinity or acidity (pH).

Furthermore, animal-based protein foods such as the ones allowed on the military diet are the type of foods that have the tendency to increase your body's acidic load, making this recommendation a little contrasting.

In addition, there is no proven research supporting the use of baking soda to decrease body fat.

The military diet which is also referred to as the 3-day diet is a restrictive periodic fasting eating plan that may promote short-term loss of weight. It is a short-term diet that may be hard and potentially not safe to sustain. The military diet which claims to help lose up to 10 pounds in 7 days (1 week) is not related or associated with the military irrespective of its name. When individuals think of the word *"military"*, they might think of a strict regimen that involves both mental and physical strength, although there is no boot camp needed with this kind of diet.

The military diet plan promotes quick and rapid loss of weight and claims that followers can lose up to 10 pounds in one week (7 days).

Nevertheless, when you lose weight quickly, some of that loss will be from water loss and muscle mass rather than body fat. The body turns to alternative energy sources for fuel anytime you drastically restrict your calorie intake.

At first, the body will start to burn glycogen, which is a form of stored carbohydrate.

* 9 7 9 8 3 3 4 9 9 1 2 8 6 *